I0695721

Table of Contents

Ankylosing spondylitis (pronounced ankle-oh-sing spon-dill-eye-tiss) is a form of arthritis that causes chronic (long-term) spine inflammation. Ankylosing spondylitis (AS) inflames the sacroiliac joints located between the base of the spine and pelvis. This inflammation, called sacroiliitis, is one of the first signs of AS. Inflammation often spreads to joints between the vertebrae, the bones that make up the spinal column. This condition is known as spondylitis.

Some people with AS experience severe, persistent back and hip pain and stiffness. Others have milder symptoms that come and go. Over time, new bone formations may fuse vertebrae sections together, making the spine rigid. This condition is called ankylosis.

5

BREAKFAST

1. Spinach Quiche

Prep Time: 30 Minutes

Cook Time: 50 Minutes

Servings: 6

Ingredients

- 1 Whole Wheat Pie Crust or your favorite pie crust dough
- 1 tablespoon extra-virgin olive oil
- 1 cup leeks white and light green parts only (about 1 small leek)
- 3 cups fresh baby spinach
- 4 large eggs
- 2 large egg whites
- 3/4 cup non-fat milk
- 1/4 cup plain non-fat Greek yogurt
- 1/4 teaspoon kosher salt
- 1/4 teaspoon black pepper

- cup reduced-fat feta cheese crumbled (4 ounces)

Instructions

1. Parbake the crust: Preheat the oven to 350 degrees F. Remove the dough from the refrigerator and place it on a well-floured surface. Working from the center, roll the dough into a 12-inch circle, then transfer it to an ungreased 9″ pie dish. With a fork, pierce rows of holes in the bottom and sides of the dough, about 1 inch apart. Bake until the crust is lightly golden, 10 to 15 minutes. Set aside to cool.

2. Prepare the filling: Heat the olive oil in a large skillet over medium-high heat. Add the leeks and sauté for 5 minutes, until tender. Add the spinach and sauté for 2 minutes. Remove from heat and set aside.

3. a mixture of creamed spinach in a pan

4. In a large bowl, whisk together the eggs, egg whites, milk, Greek yogurt, salt, and pepper. Set aside.

5. beaten eggs with milk in a mixing bowl

6. Spoon the spinach and leek mixture into the bottom of the crust, then sprinkle the feta over the top.

7. cooked spinach with feta in an empty pie shell

8. Gently pour in the egg mixture.

9 a unbaked pie crust filled with eggs, spinach and feta ready to bake

10 Bake the quiche for 45 to 55 minutes, until eggs are set in the center and puffed slightly and the crust is golden brown. Let the quiche cool on a wire rack for 10 minutes. Slice and serve warm or at room temperature.

Prep Time: 10 Minutes

Cook Time: 10 Minutes

Servings: 8

Ingredients

- large eggs
- 1 tablespoon milk
- 1/2 teaspoon salt
- 1/2 teaspoon garlic powder
- 1/2 teaspoon black pepper
- 1/2 tablespoon extra-virgin olive oil
- 5 cups lightly packed fresh spinach roughly torn or chopped (about 4 ounces)
- 1 can reduced-sodium white beans (15 ounces) , such as, Great Northern, or white kidney, rinsed and drained (I typically use cannellini)
- 1 1/2 cups freshly grated cheese such as cheddar, Swiss, mozzarella, or another similar melty cheese; I love sharp white cheddar (about 5 ounces)
- 8 whole wheat tortillas medium taco size, about 7 inches

Instructions

1 In a large bowl, whisk together the eggs, milk, salt, garlic powder, and pepper. Set aside.

2 Add the olive oil to a large nonstick skillet over medium heat until it is hot and shimmers. Swirl to coat the pan, then add the spinach and cook, stirring often, until it begins to wilt, about 1 minute. Add the beans, reduce the heat to medium low, then carefully pour in the eggs. With a rubber spatula, cook the eggs low and slow, using the spatula to move them around the pan often. Continue cooking until the eggs are scrambled and just set, about 5 minutes. Taste and season with additional salt or pepper as desired. Remove from the heat. (If freezing the quesadillas, let the filling cool completely.)

3 Assemble the quesadillas by sprinkling a tortilla with one-eighth of the shredded cheese, leaving a small border all the way around the edge. Spoon one-eighth of the egg mixture on top, then fold the tortilla in half. Repeat with the remaining tortillas.

4 To Cook Immediately

5 Carefully wipe out the skillet. Increase the heat to medium and lightly coat the skillet with nonstick spray (or brush with a bit of additional olive oil). Cook

the assembled quesadillas on both sides until golden and the cheese is melted, about 5 to 6 minutes total. Cut into wedges and serve warm.

6 To Freeze

7 Let the egg filling cool completely to room temperature. Once cooled, form the quesadillas as directed above, then wrap each assembled quesadilla individually in plastic wrap. Arrange the quesadillas in a single layer on a baking sheet or similar flat surface that will fit in your freezer. Place the sheet in the freezer until the quesadillas are firm, then transfer them to a freezer bag or airtight container. Freeze for up to 2 months. To cook from frozen, remove the plastic wrap and warm the quesadilla in the microwave for 2 to 3 minutes until heated through. Alternatively, you can let them thaw overnight in the refrigerator and cook in a skillet as directed above.

Prep Time: 10 Minutes

Cook Time: 40 Minutes

Servings: 4

Ingredients

For the Vegetables:

- 2 tablespoons extra-virgin olive oil or melted coconut oil, divided
- 1 small red onion cut into 1-inch wedges
- 2 large sweet potatoes scrubbed with skins on, halved lengthwise
- 2 teaspoons chili powder divided
- 3/4 teaspoon salt divided
- 3/4 teaspoon black pepper divided
- 1 small head broccoli or cauliflower
- 1 small bunch kale large stems removed

For the Dressing:

- 3 tablespoons lemon juice about 1 small lemon
- 3 tablespoons tahini or swap natural almond butter
- 1 clove garlic minced

- 1/2-1 teaspoon ground cumin
- 1/4 teaspoon salt
- 4 hard-boiled eggs or soft-boiled, see recipe notes

Instructions

1   Place a rack in the center of your oven and preheat the oven to 400 degrees F. Liberally coat a rimmed baking sheet with nonstick spray and set aside.

2   Place the onions and sweet potatoes on the baking sheet, turning the sweet potatoes cut sides up. Drizzle with 2 teaspoons olive oil, making sure the flesh of the sweet potatoes is well coated. Sprinkle with 1 teaspoon chili powder, 1/4 teaspoon salt, and 1/4 teaspoon pepper. Rub and toss to coat, and then arrange on the baking sheet. Bake for 10 minutes.

3   While the sweet potatoes cook, chop the broccoli or cauliflower into florets (you should have about 5 cups total). Remove the baking sheet from the oven and flip the sweet potatoes so that they are cut sides down. Push the sweet potatoes and onions to one side and add the cauliflower or broccoli to the open side of the pan. Drizzle with 2 teaspoons olive oil and sprinkle with 1/4 teaspoon salt, 1/4 teaspoon pepper, and the

remaining 1 teaspoon chili powder. Carefully toss to coat, and then return the baking sheet to the oven. The pan will be very crowded, and the veggies will overlap somewhat. Return to the oven and bake for an additional 20 to 25 minutes, until the sweet potatoes are soft and the other vegetables are crisp-tender.

4 Remove the sheet pan from the oven and place the kale on top of the vegetables. Drizzle the kale with the remaining 2 teaspoons olive oil and sprinkle with the remaining 1/4 teaspoon salt and 1/4 teaspoon pepper. Lightly rub the kale to coat, and then arrange the kale in a single layer over the whole pan. Return the pan to the oven and bake for 5 additional minutes, until the kale is very lightly crisp and softened. Remove the whole pan from the oven and set it aside to cool.

5 While vegetables finish roasting, prepare the dressing: Add the lemon juice, tahini, garlic, cumin, and salt in a small mixing bowl. Add 2 tablespoons hot water. Whisk to combine. Taste and add additional salt and up to 1/2 teaspoon additional cumin as desired.

6 To serve: Once the vegetables are cool enough to handle, cut the sweet potatoes into bite-size pieces. Roughly chop the kale. Divide the vegetables among serving bowls. Slice the hardboiled eggs in half and

place 2 halves on top of each bowl. Drizzle with tahini dressing and enjoy immediately.

Prep Time: 30 Minutes

Cook Time: 15 Minutes

Servings: 8

Ingredients

- Nonstick cooking spray
- strips bacon cooked
- 2 1/2 pounds russet potatoes
- 1 tablespoon extra-virgin olive oil
- 1 tablespoon all-purpose flour
- 1 1/4 teaspoons salt
- 1 teaspoon garlic powder
- 1/2 teaspoon black pepper
- 1/2 cup freshly grated sharp cheddar cheese about 2 ounces—OK to swap reduced fat, but do not use fat free
- 3 tablespoons chopped chives or green onion
- Nonfat plain Greek yogurt or sour cream (for serving, optional)

Instructions

1 If necessary, cook the bacon according to one of my easy methods listed below. Once cool, dice into small pieces.

2 Increase the oven temperature to 425 degrees F. Scrub and peel the potatoes. Place potatoes in a large pot and cover with 1 inch of cold water. Bring to a simmer over medium heat and cook for 6 minutes (the potatoes should be about halfway cooked). Drain and let cool for 15 minutes.

3 parboiled potatoes cooling in a fine mesh strainer

4 Once cooled, grate the potatoes into a large bowl.

5 cooled grated potatoes in a glass bowl to make homemade tater tots

6 Add the olive oil, flour, salt, garlic powder, and black pepper. Gently combine by hand so that the ingredients are as evenly distributed as possible.

7 adding flour and spices to a bowl of shredded potatoes for tater tots in oven

8 Add the bacon, cheese, and chives.

9 a glass bowl of shredded potatoes for tater tots with cheese and bacon and onions

10 Stir to combine.

11 a mixture of uncooked tater tots ingredients ready to shape

12 Generously coat two 24-cup mini muffin tins with nonstick spray, or make the tots in two batches. With a spoon, scoop about one heaping tablespoon of the potato mixture into each muffin cavity, then with your fingers, press each scoop flat.

13 a mini muffin pan filled with tater tots without egg

14 Bake until the potatoes are brown at the edges, about 15 minutes, then remove from the oven and coat the tops with cooking spray. With a small offset spatula or table knife, flip each tot. Coat tops with nonstick spray once more, then return the pan to the oven and bake until browned, 12 to 15 additional minutes until golden brown. Let cool in the pan for 2 minutes, then serve with Greek yogurt or sour cream.

15 A plate of golden brown tater tots with cheese and bacon topped with Greek yogurt and green onions

Prep Time: 5 Minutes

Cook Time: 15 Minutes

Servings: 2-3

Ingredients

- 2 teaspoons extra-virgin olive oil
- 1 small red onion diced (about 1 cup)
- 3 cloves garlic minced (about 1 tablespoon)
- 1 can reduced-sodium chickpeas (15 ounces), rinsed and drained
- 1 jar good-quality tomato pasta sauce (24 ounces)
- 1 teaspoon dried oregano
- 1 teaspoon salt
- 1/4 teaspoon red pepper flakes
- 5 ounces baby spinach
- 4 large eggs
- 1/2 cup Parmesan cheese freshly grated
- fresh basil chopped
- Baguette slices for serving

Instructions

1   Place a rack in the center of your oven and preheat the oven to 375 degrees F.

2   Heat the olive oil in a large, ovenproof, nonstick skillet over medium-high. Add the onion and cook, stirring often, until the onion is translucent, about 3 minutes. Add the garlic and cook just until fragrant, about 30 seconds.

3   Stir in the chickpeas, tomato sauce, oregano, salt, and red pepper flakes. Bring to a simmer and let cook until slightly thickened, about 3 minutes.

4   Stir in the spinach a few handfuls at a time, letting it wilt.

5   With the back of a spoon, make 4 indentations in the sauce. Crack one egg inside of each, then sprinkle the Parmesan cheese over the whole dish.

6   Carefully transfer the pan to the oven. Bake until the egg whites are set but the yolks are still soft, 10 to 12 minutes. Remove from the oven and sprinkle with fresh basil. Serve hot with baguette slices.

Prep Time: 5 Minutes

Cook Time: 15 Minutes

Servings: 12

Ingredients

For the Muffins:

- 1 cup whole wheat flour
- 3/4 cup old fashioned rolled oats
- 1/2 cup oat flour (or 1/2 cup plus 2 tablespoons oats finely ground in a food processor)
- 1 tablespoon baking powder
- 1 1/2 teaspoons ground cinnamon
- 1/2 teaspoon salt
- 1/4 teaspoon ground nutmeg
- 1 cup non-fat milk plus 2 tablespoons
- 1/2 cup pure maple syrup
- 1/4 cup coconut oil melted and cooled, or substitute canola oil or melted and cooled unsalted butter
- 2 large eggs at room temperature
- 1 teaspoon vanilla extract

For the Crumb Topping:

- 1 tablespoon cold unsalted butter cut into small pieces
- 3 tablespoons flour
- 1 tablespoon brown sugar
- 1/2 teaspoon ground cinnamon

Instructions

1. Preheat the oven to 400 degrees F. Lightly grease a standard 12-cup muffin tin or line with paper liners and set aside.
2. In a large bowl, stir together the whole wheat flour, oats, oat flour, baking powder, cinnamon, salt, and nutmeg.
3. dry ingredients in a mixing bowl for healthy oat muffins
4. In a separate bowl, whisk together the milk, maple syrup, oil (or butter), eggs, and vanilla. Make a well in the center of the dry ingredients, then pour the wet ingredients into the center.
5. milk, maple syrup, and eggs in a mixing bowl with a whisk

6. By hand, stir the batter gently, just until combined (it will be somewhat lumpy). Divide the batter evenly between the prepared muffin cups.

7. A bowl of healthy oat muffin batter in a mixing bowl

For the crumb topping:

1. In a small bowl, quickly rub the butter, flour, brown sugar, and cinnamon together with your fingers until fine crumbs form. Sprinkle over each unbaked muffin.

2. healthy muffin batter topped with crumb topping unbaked in a muffin pan

3. Bake the muffins until golden brown and a toothpick in the center comes out clean, 18-20 minutes. Allow the muffins to cool in the pan for 5 minutes, then gently remove to a wire rack to cool completely.

4. freshly-baked healthy oatmeal muffins no banana

Prep Time: 40 Minutes

Cook Time: 55 Minutes

Servings: 6

Ingredients

- dates, pitted and soaked
- 1 large banana, ripe
- 1 cup peanut, almond, or other nut butter
- 1 scoop protein powder (unflavored, vanilla, or chocolate)
- 1/4 cup shelled hemp seeds
- 1/4 cup chia seeds
- 2 1/4 cups gluten-free rolled oats

Optional add-ins:

- 1 tsp. cinnamon, or
- 1-2 tsp. cocoa powder (if you aren't using chocolate protein powder)
- Pinch of salt

Instructions

1. Soak dates in enough water to cover for 1-2 hours before using (this will help them blend easier).

2. Drain the dates thoroughly, and add them to the bowl of your food processor. Add the banana, and pulse to a smooth paste, scraping down the sides as needed.

3. Add the nut butter, protein powder, hemp seeds, chia seeds, and any add-ins you like. Pulse to combine – the mixture will become very thick and may slow down your food processor.

4. Remove the mixture to a large bowl, and add in the oats. Using a flexible rubber spatula, fold the oats into the nut butter paste. You'll think there's no way for so many oats to incorporate in, but just keep folding it and soon enough it will come together.

5. Line one 8x8inch square baking pan with parchment paper, and scoop the mixture into it. Spread it as evenly as you can with the back of a spatula, then fold the edges of the parchment over the top (or cover with an additional sheet of parchment). Press down along the top to smooth out any remaining bumps, and place in the freezer for 2-3 hours, or overnight, or until thoroughly frozen.

6   Remove from freezer, unwrap, and slice into bars. I like to make 6 large, meal-sized bars, but feel free to cut them smaller. Once cut, seal bars in a zip-top freezer bag and store in the freezer indefinitely. You may want to separate bars with parchment to keep them from sticking.

7   When you want to feel perfectly full, incredibly satisfied, and thoroughly satiated – remove one bar from the freezer, and enjoy. Fresh from the freezer they are firm, but chewy. If left out to thaw, they become quite soft and sticky. If you wanted to prevent this, it may be possible to dip the bars in chocolate to create a shell on the outside... but I've never tried.

Prep Time: 20 Minutes

Cook Time: 25 Minutes

Servings: 4-6

Ingredients

- 2 Cups all-purpose flour (or a mix of whole wheat, or buckwheat)
- 2 Cups whole milk or milk substitute, warm (if using 50/50 whole wheat flour, increase by 2 TBSP – if using 100% whole wheat, increase by 1/4 cup)
- 1/2 Cup water, warm (110-115f. – if the water is too hot it may inhibit bacteria growth, rather than promote it. I suggest an instant read thermometer)
- 2 tsp. active dry yeast powder
- 4 Tbsp (or half a stick) unsalted butter, melted
- 1-2 tsp. sugar, depending on your preference
- 1 tsp. salt
- 2 large eggs
- 1/4 tsp. baking soda

Optional:

- 1/2 tsp. vanilla extract

Optional:

- 1/2 tsp. almond extract (or other flavor)

Optional:

- Any additional add-ins, such as nuts, chocolate chips, fruit, cinnamon or other spices, etc....

Instructions

1. In a large bowl (bigger than you think you'll need, the yeast will expand) sprinkle the yeast over 1/2 cup warm water. After a minute or so, add the sugar. Let this sit for 5-10 minutes so the yeast can dissolve a little and start doing its thing.

2. Once the yeast has rested, add the melted butter, warm milk, flour, and salt. Mix thoroughly until smooth (a whisk works well, here).

3. Cover loosely with plastic wrap, or a clean towel, and let sit at room temp. overnight. If it's particularly hot the batter can be stored in the fridge. If making the waffle mix more than one night in advance, leave un-chilled for the first night and then store in the fridge for up to three more days.

4   When ready to use, preheat your waffle iron, and preheat oven to 200f.

5   Whisk eggs in a small bowl, then sprinkle in the baking soda and whisk to combine – be sure there are no lumps of baking soda remaining. Pour egg mixture into the batter and whisk until smooth.

6   Depending on your iron, you may need 1/2-1 cup batter per waffle. The batter will be very thin, so just pour into the center of your iron and let it spread. Cook according to manufacturer's instructions, or to desired done-ness.

7   Transfer finished waffles directly to the rack of the oven to keep warm and fresh until ready to be eaten.

8   Serve with your favorite toppings, or try my recipe for a yogurt fruit spread!

Prep Time: 20 Minutes

Cook Time: 25 Minutes

Servings: 4-6

Ingredients

- 1 lb. Bacon
- 1/2 cup brown sugar
- 2 cups pancake mix (homemade or Bisquick style)
- 2 cups of your favorite beer, alcoholic or non, separated (I used Founder's – a local brewery I like. The Porter I chose is very dark, hoppy, and has undertones of coffee and chocolate. It was a great pairing with the salty bacon and sweet syrup. Guinness would work well, too, or whatever kind of beer you like.)
- 2 eggs
- 1 – 2 cups maple syrup (I like grade B because it's darker and sweeter, but use what you have/what you prefer)

Instructions

1. Preheat oven to 350f.

2. Line a cookie sheet with foil, and set inside of that a wire rack or oven grill grate. Lay the bacon flat, in a single layer, on top of the rack and bake for 10 minutes.

3. Take the bacon out, and sprinkle evenly with half of the brown sugar – bake for 10 minutes more.

4. Remove the bacon again, and turn each piece over. Sprinkle this side with the second half of brown sugar, and bake for another 10-15 minutes, until nice and golden.

5. Remove from the oven and let cool completely before crumbling into pieces.

6. Get your griddle or skillet heating up – medium-high should do the trick.

7. In a large bowl, whisk together the pancake mix, 1 cup beer, and eggs. If it's too thick add more beer, too thin add more mix. Stir in the bacon.

8. Grease your griddle (oil, butter, shortening, spray...) and ladle/scoop/pour your batter into whatever size pancakes you want.

9. Cook on one side until bubbles appear on the top and the edges begin to look dry, then flip.

10 In a small saucepan, combine the remaining beer with 1 cup of maple syrup. Stir, and bring to a simmer. Reduce heat to low. If it's too thin, or too much beer for your taste, adjust by adding more maple syrup. If you don't want the extra layer of beer, you can skip this whole step and just warm up your maple syrup.

11 Serve hot.

Prep Time: 20 Minutes

Cook Time: 25 Minutes

Servings: 8

Ingredients

- 3 cups riced cauliflower from about 1 ¼ pounds or ½ medium head cauliflower or thawed frozen riced cauliflower
- 1 large egg
- 3/4 cup shredded sharp cheddar cheese
- ¼ cup grated Parmesan
- ½ teaspoon salt
- ¼ teaspoon ground black pepper
- ¼ teaspoon garlic powder

- ¼ teaspoon onion powder
- ¼ teaspoon smoked paprika or 1/8 teaspoon cayenne pepper
- Non-stick cooking spray

Instructions

1. Place racks in the center and upper third of your oven. Preheat the oven to 400 degrees F. Generously coat a rimmed baking sheet with nonstick spray or line with parchment paper.
2. Place the cauliflower rice in a microwave-safe bowl. Microwave on high, uncovered, for 2 minutes.
3. Finely chopped vegetables in a bowl
4. Spread the cauliflower onto a clean, dry kitchen towel and let cool for 5 minutes; keep the cauliflower fairly centered on the towel.
5. Bring the sides of the towel up and around the cauliflower to make a purse. Squeeze as much moisture out of the cauliflower as possible. The drier it is, the crispier the cauliflower hash browns will be.
6. Water being squeezed from riced cauliflower
7. To a large, dry mixing bowl, add the egg. Lightly beat it with a fork, then stir in the cheddar, Parmesan, salt,

black pepper, garlic powder, onion powder, and smoked paprika.

8   Cheese, eggs, and spices in a bowl

9   Add the cauliflower to the bowl and mix to thoroughly combine.

10 A mixing bowl with ingredients for cauliflower hash browns

11 Divide the cauliflower mixture into 8 equal portions. Working one portion at a time, squeeze the portion firmly into a ball with your hands, then gently flatten with your hands to shape into patties that are about 1/2-inch thick. Arrange the patties evenly on the baking sheet, leaving at least 1 inch of space between each.

12 Vegetable patties on a baking sheet

13 Bake on the center rack until lightly browned and set, about 15 minutes, rotating the pan 180 degrees halfway through.

14 Turn the broiler to low. Transfer the pan to the upper-third rack and bake until crispy on top, about 5 minutes. Watch very carefully so that the hash browns do not burn.

15 Let cool on the baking sheet for 5 minutes to set. Enjoy hot.

11. Butternut Squash Apple Soup

Prep Time: 20 Minutes

Cook Time: 40 Minutes

Servings: 8

Ingredients

For the Soup:

- 2 tablespoons olive oil
- 2 medium yellow onions chopped (about 3 cups total)
- 2 large butternut squash about 5 pounds total, peeled and diced into chunks
- 4 medium apples (or 3 large) I like using a mix of sweet apples such as McIntosh or Golden Delicious and tart such as Granny Smith or Cortland, peeled, cored and roughly diced
- 3-4 cups low sodium chicken stock divided
- 1 1/4 teaspoon kosher salt
- 1/2 teaspoon freshly grated nutmeg
- 1/4 teaspoon black pepper
- 1/4 teaspoon cayenne pepper

For the Sage Parmesan Croutons:

- cups sourdough cubes or whole grain bread cubes(1-inch cut) use a hearty, crusty loaf—you'll need about 6 thick slices total
- 3 tablespoons olive oil
- 2 tablespoons minced fresh sage
- 1/2 teaspoon kosher salt
- 3 tablespoons freshly grated parmesan

Instructions

1. Preheat your oven to 375 degrees. In a large, deep stockpot or Dutch oven, heat the olive oil over low. Add the onions and cook until very tender, about 15 to 20 minutes, stirring occasionally.
2. Double your deposit & hit the targets
3. While the onions cook, cut and peel the squash and apples. Add them to the pot, then add 2 cups of the stock. Bring the pot to a boil, reduce the heat to low, then cover, and cook until the squash and apples are very soft, about 20 to 30 minutes depending upon how larger you cut your squash and apple pieces (smaller pieces will cook more quickly).

4   Meanwhile, prepare the croutons. Place the bread cubes on a large baking sheet. Drizzle with olive oil, sprinkle with sage and salt, then toss to coat. Spread the cubes in a single layer, then bake until lightly crisp and brown, 10 to 12 minutes, tossing once halfway through. Sprinkle with Parmesan cheese, toss to coat, then set aside until ready to serve.

5   Once the apples and squash in the soup pot are tender, puree the soup with an immersion blender or carefully transfer it to a food processor fitted with a steel blade to puree in batches. Return soup to the pot once complete. Add 1 cup of the remaining chicken stock, then stir, adding a bit more stock as needed to reach your desired consistency (the soup will thicken somewhat when stored). Leave the texture fairly thick and rich. Stir in the salt, nutmeg, black pepper, and cayenne. Taste and add a bit more salt and pepper as desired. Serve hot, topped with sage croutons.

Prep Time: 10 Minutes

Cook Time: 15 Minutes

Servings: 8

Ingredients

- 4 whole wheat English muffins split
- 1/2 tablespoon extra virgin olive oil
- 3/4 cup prepared pizza sauce tomato, pesto, or alfredo; whichever your family likes! (We use tomato)
- Tiny Pinch salt
- Pinch black pepper
- 1 cup shredded part-skim mozzarella cheese or cheddar cheese, provolone, or any cheese you like
- 1/2 teaspoon Italian seasoning
- Toppings of choice such as mini pepperonis (or regular pepperonis, quartered), or sautéed veggies, such as spinach or mushrooms
- Thinly sliced fresh basil optional for serving

Instructions

1. Preheat the oven to 400 degrees F. Line a baking sheet with parchment paper.

2. Arrange the English muffin halves cut side up onto a baking sheet. Lightly drizzle with olive oil. Place in the oven and toast until barely golden, about 4 minutes.

3. Spoon 1 1/2 tablespoons pizza sauce over each one, using the back of a spoon to spread it evenly. Sprinkle with salt and pepper. Top with mozzarella cheese and Italian seasoning. Add any desired toppings.

4. Bake for 10 minutes, until the cheese is melted and the muffins are browned on the edges. Top with fresh basil. Enjoy hot.

Prep Time: 10 Minutes

Cook Time: 15 Minutes

Servings: 4

Ingredients

- 1 pound sirloin top round steak, or flank steak
- 1/2 teaspoon baking soda
- tablespoons water divided
- ounces long noodles such as whole grain spaghetti or whole grain fettuccine, soba noodles, or udon noodles
- 1/4 cup reduced sodium soy sauce plus additional to taste
- 1/4 cup hoisin sauce
- 4 cloves garlic minced or grated (about 1 heaping tablespoon)
- 1 tablespoon finely chopped fresh ginger
- 1/2 teaspoon crushed red pepper flakes plus additional to taste
- 1 tablespoon canola oil or peanut or grapeseed oil
- 2 medium carrots peeled and cut into thin coins

- 1 head broccoli cut into small florets (about 3 cups), or 3 cups thinly sliced cabbage

- 1 red bell pepper cored and thinly sliced

- 1 8-ounce can sliced water chestnuts, drained

- 4 green onions thinly sliced divided

- 2 teaspoons toasted sesame oil optional

Instructions

1 For easier slicing, place the beef in the freezer for 15 minutes to firm up. Cut the beef across the grain into very thin (1/4-inch or smaller) slices. Cut any long slices in half cross wise (each strip should be around 3 inches or so long).

2 Place the beef in a medium bowl. In a small bowl, stir together the baking soda and 2 tablespoons of the water. Pour over the beef and toss to coat. Let sit 5 minutes (this helps to tenderize it).

3 Meanwhile, in a large pot of salted water, cook the noodles just until al dente. Drain and rinse under cool water. Set aside.

4 In a small bowl or larger liquid measuring cup, stir together the soy sauce, hoisin, garlic, ginger, and red pepper flakes. Keep handy near the stove.

5   soy, garlic, and ginger sauce mix in cup for beef lo mein recipe

6   In a wok or large, nonstick skillet, heat the oil over medium high. Add the beef and cook until crisp on the outside but still pink on the inside, about 3 minutes. The beef will give off liquid, which is fine. Stir in 1 tablespoon of the sauce and let cook 30 seconds. With a large spoon, scoop the beef onto a plate (any cooking juices left behind will cook away).

7   sliced beef in a skillet for beef lo mein

8   Add the carrots, broccoli, and bell pepper. Cook until crisp-tender, about 2 minutes. Stir in the remaining 4 tablespoons (1/4 cup) of water and let the vegetables steam until the broccoli turns bright green and most of the liquid has cooked away, about 2 minutes more.

9   broccoli and vegetables for beef lo mein in a skillet

10 Stir in the water chestnuts, half of the green onions, and 2 tablespoons of the soy sauce mixture and let cook 30 additional seconds.

11 Reduce the heat to medium. Add the noodles and beef and pour the remaining soy sauce mixture over the top. With tongs, stir and toss until the noodles are heated through.

12 Drizzle the sesame oil over the top (if using) and sprinkle on the remaining green onion. Toss to combine. Enjoy!

Prep Time: 10 Minutes

Cook Time: 0 Minutes

Servings: 4

Ingredients

- 1/2 cup dry-packed sun-dried tomatoes or oil packed sun-dried tomatoes
- 1/3 cup homemade Caesar dressing or Caesar dressing of choice, divided
- 1 teaspoon Worcestershire sauce optional for a more intense flavor
- 2 1/2 cups cooked diced or shredded chicken breast about 2 medium breasts;
- 1 romaine lettuce heart chopped (about 4 cups)
- 1/3 cup shredded Parmesan cheese (no green can please!)
- 1/4 teaspoon salt
- 1/4 teaspoon ground black pepper
- 4 whole wheat wraps or flatbreads such as pita, naan, or tortillas

Instructions

1. If using dry-packed sun-dried tomatoes, place them in a small bowl and cover with hot water to rehydrate. Let sit for a few minutes while you prepare the rest of the ingredients, then drain. If using oil-packed sun-dried tomatoes, simply pat them dry.

2. Place the Caesar dressing in a medium bowl. Stir together with 1 teaspoon Worcestershire sauce. Add the chicken, romaine, sun-dried tomatoes, Parmesan, salt, and black pepper. Toss to coat in the dressing.

3. A bowl of salad with meat

4. For each chicken Caesar wrap, lay your wrap down on a work surface. Pile each wrap with 1/4 of the chicken Caesar filling. Roll snugly, tucking in two opposing sides to keep the filling from falling out. If desired, slice in half. Enjoy immediately or wrap in foil, parchment paper, or plastic wrap and refrigerate for up to 4 hours.

Prep Time: 10 Minutes

Cook Time: 45 Minutes

Servings: 6

Ingredients

- 2 tablespoons mild curry powder
- 2 teaspoons ground allspice
- 1 tablespoon brown sugar
- ½-1½ teaspoons hot chilli powder (or more, for a spicier version)
- ½ teaspoon ground turmeric
- 800 grams skinless, boneless Rangitikei chicken thighs
- 2 teaspoons sea salt
- 2 tablespoons olive oil
- 1 tablespoon butter
- 1 large onion, thinly sliced
- 3 cloves garlic, crushed
- 2 tablespoons grated fresh ginger
- 4 sprigs thyme
- 3 bay leaves

- 1½ cups chicken stock
- 1½ cups coconut cream
- 2 tablespoons soy sauce
- smallish red potatoes, halved
- 2 medium carrots, sliced on the diagonal
- 2 jalapeno chillies

Instructions

1 Combine the curry powder, allspice, sugar, chilli powder and turmeric in a small bowl. Halve the chicken thighs and place in a large bowl. Sprinkle with 2 tablespoons of the spice mix and the sea salt and turn to coat well. Reserve the remaining spice mix.

2 Heat the oil and butter in a large, deep frying pan or saucepan over a medium heat. Cook the chicken in batches for 1 minute each side, until golden, then transfer to a plate. Don't let the spices catch and burn.

3 Add the onion, garlic, ginger, 2 sprigs thyme and the bay leaves to the pan and cook for 5 minutes, adding a splash of water if the pan is too dry. Stir in the reserved spice mix and cook for

4 30 seconds.

5   Stir in the stock, coconut cream and soy, then add the potatoes and carrots. Bring to the boil, cover and simmer for 20 minutes.

6   Add the chicken, jalapeños and remaining thyme and bring back up to the boil. Reduce the heat and simmer gently for about 25 minutes with the lid slightly ajar, or until the chicken is fully cooked and the vegetables are tender. Serve with lots of hot, cooked rice or warm flatbreads.

Prep Time: 50 Minutes

Cook Time: 45 Minutes

Servings: 4-5

Ingredients

- 500 grams frozen squid tubes
- ½ cup plain flour
- ½ cup semolina flour
- ⅓ cup fine polenta
- 2 teaspoons garlic powder
- 2 teaspoons chipotle powder
- 1 teaspoon table salt
- vegetable oil, for frying
- 2 cloves garlic, finely sliced
- 1 red chilli, sliced
- olive oil
- finely grated zest ½ lime, plus juice to serve
- sea salt
- good-quality egg mayonnaise, to serve

Instructions

1. Defrost and rinse the squid tubes, then cut into shapes. I like to do a combination of rings and lattice-scored rectangles.
2. In a large bowl, combine the flours, polenta, garlic powder, chipotle powder and salt.
3. Heat 5cm of vegetable oil to 180°C in a large saucepan. Dredge the squid in the flour mixture and fry in batches until golden and crisp. Remove with a slotted spoon and drain on a tray lined with paper towels.
4. In a small frying pan, briefly fry the garlic and chilli in a little olive oil until the garlic is just starting to colour.
5. In a large bowl, toss together the squid, lime zest, fried garlic and chilli and sea salt to taste.
6. Serve hot with mayonnaise and a squeeze of lime juice.

Prep Time: 25 Minutes

Cook Time: 30 Minutes

Servings: 2

Ingredients

- 400 grams centre cut salmon fillet, skin off
- 2 teaspoons whole cumin seeds
- 1 teaspoon smoked paprika
- ¼ teaspoon ground turmeric
- 2 tablespoons olive oil
- sea salt and ground pepper
- 3 medium zucchini, very thinly sliced
- To serve
- 200 grams purchased babaghanoush
- ¼ cup purchased chimichurri
- 2 tablespoons purchased dukkah
- Equipment: 4 x 20cm thin metal skewers.

Instructions

1 Cut the salmon into 12 pieces. Combine the spices and oil in a large bowl and season well. Add the salmon and turn to coat. Spread the zucchini into a single layer and season. Thread a few slices at a time onto the skewers along with the salmon. Heat a little oil in a large frying pan and, when hot, cook the skewers for about 1½ minutes each side, or until cooked to your liking.

2 To serve: Spread the babaghanoush over two plates. Top each with two skewers, then spoon over the chimichurri and scatter with dukkah. Add a final drizzle of olive oil.

Prep Time: 20 Minutes

Cook Time: 30 Minutes

Servings: 4

Ingredients

- 1 1/2 pound center-cut, skin-on side of salmon
- 1 tablespoon olive oil
- 1 teaspoon ground cumin divided
- 3/4 teaspoon kosher salt divided
- 1/2 teaspoon black pepper
- 1/2 teaspoon ground oregano divided
- 1/2 small red onion finely chopped
- 1/3 cup nonfat plain Greek yogurt
- Zest of 2 mediums lemon about 2 teaspoons
- tablespoons fresh lemon juice
- 1 clove minced or grated garlic
- 2 mini cucumbers or 1/2 English cucumber, cut into 1/2-inch dice (about 1 1/2 cups)
- 1/2 cup crumbled feta
- 1/4 cup toasted sliced almonds
- 1/4 cup currents raisins, or golden raisins

- 1/4 cup chopped fresh dill
- 1/4 cup chopped fresh cilantro

Instructions

1. Preheat the oven to 400 degrees F. Line a baking dish large enough to hold the salmon with a sheet of parchment paper.
2. Place the salmon in the pan and with paper towels, pat dry. Drizzle with the olive oil and sprinkle with 1/2 teaspoon cumin, 1/2 teaspoon salt, pepper, and 1/4 teaspoon oregano. Rub to evenly coat the salmon. Bake for 14 to 18 minutes, until the salmon reaches an internal temperature of 145 degrees F on an instant read thermometer (I typically remove the salmon a few degrees early and let the carryover cooking finish the rest). The salmon should no longer be raw-looking in the center and flake easily with a fork. Let cool to room temperature.
3. Salmon in a baking dish
4. While the salmon roasts, place the red onion in a bowl and cover with cold water. Set aside to soak (this removes some of the onion's harsh bite without losing its flavor).

5   Prepare the dressing: In a small mixing bowl, stir together the yogurt, lemon zest, lemon juice, and remaining 1/4 teaspoon cumin, 1/4 teaspoon salt, and 1/4 teaspoon oregano.

6   Dressing being mixed in a bowl

7   Flake the salmon in chunky pieces into a large serving bowl (discard the skin).

8   Salmon pieces on a plate

9   Add the cucumber, feta, currants, dill, and cilantro.

10 Raisins, almonds, and cheese being added to a bowl

11 Drain the red onion, then add it to the bowl.

12 Pour the dressing over the top.

13 Ingredients being mixed with dressing in a bowl

14 Gently stir to combine. Taste and season with additional salt and pepper as desired (I add an extra pinch of each). Serve chilled or at room temperature as a wrap (or lettuce wrap), sandwich, on toast, over greens, or mixed with couscous.

15 Scrumptious salmon salad in a bowl

Prep Time: 20 Minutes

Cook Time: 30 Minutes

Servings: 6-8

Ingredients

- kilograms beef cheeks
- 2 tablespoons olive oil
- 80 grams pancetta, chopped
- 1 onion, finely chopped
- cloves garlic, crushed
- 1 tablespoon finely chopped fresh rosemary
- 2 tablespoons finely chopped fresh oregano
- 2 tablespoons tomato paste
- 2½ cups red wine
- 1 cup passata
- 2 teaspoons caster sugar
- sea salt and ground pepper
- 1 cup sunblush tomatoes, roughly chopped
- large black olives

To serve

- hot, cooked pappardelle
- Salsa Verde
- 1 cup freshly grated parmesan

Instructions

1 Trim any sinew from the beef cheeks and cut them in half. Heat the oil in a large casserole dish and, in batches, sear the beef for a few minutes on all sides. Remove from the pan and set aside. Don't wash the pan.

2 Add the pancetta to the pan and cook over a medium-high heat for 3-4 minutes, then reduce the heat and add the onion, garlic, rosemary and oregano. Cook for 10 minutes, until the onion is softened but not coloured. Add the tomato paste, wine, passata and sugar and stir to combine. Season to taste and bring to the boil.

3 Add the beef cheeks back to the pan and bring to the boil. Reduce the heat to low, cover and cook on the stovetop for 3 hours. Stir in the tomatoes and olives and cook for a further 1 hour. Remove and shred the beef cheeks, then add them back to the sauce.

4   TO SERVE: Serve over hot pappardelle and top with a
    spoonful of Salsa Verde and parmesan.

Prep Time: 20 Minutes

Cook Time: 40 Minutes

Servings: 4

Ingredients

For the Buddha Bowl and Quinoa:

- 3/4 cup uncooked quinoa
- 3/4 pound cut broccoli florets
- 3/4 pound cut cauliflower florets about 1/2 medium-sized head, cut into slightly smaller pieces than the broccoli
- 1 medium red onion cut into 1/2-inch rings, rings mostly separated but still left "chunky" (no need to split every layer)
- tablespoons extra virgin olive oil
- 1/2 teaspoon kosher salt plus additional for cooking the quinoa
- 1/4 teaspoon black pepper
- 1 block extra firm tofu (12 to 14-ounces) (do not use firm or silken), removed from packaged and pressed dry

- 2 small ripe Hass avocados
- Optional for serving: Sliced cucumbers and toasted almonds or pistachios, additional fresh mint and parsley

For the Tahini Dressing:

- 1/2 cup tahini well stirred
- 1/4 cup freshly squeezed lemon juice about 2 large lemons
- 1 1/2 cups lightly packed fresh mint leaves about 1 of the herb packs
- 1/2 cup lightly packed fresh parsley leaves
- 3/4 teaspoon kosher salt
- 1/4 teaspoon black pepper

Instructions

1   Bring 1 1/2 cups of water to a boil. Add 1/2 teaspoon kosher salt and the quinoa. Return to boil, cover, then reduce heat and simmer for 12 minutes, until most of the liquid is absorbed. Remove from the heat, fluff with a fork, then recover and let stand for 15 minutes. (This is the cooking process for the brand of quinoa I

use. Check the package of your quinoa and cook according to its directions.) Set cooked quinoa aside.

2   Place a rack in the upper and lower thirds of your oven and preheat your oven to 400 degrees F. While the quinoa cooks and the oven preheats, place the tofu between two kitchen towels and set it on a plate. Place a second plate on top, then press firmly to press out as much water from the tofu as you can, changing out the towels as needed. Dice into 3/4-inch cubes, then spread in a single layer on a baking sheet lined with parchment paper.

3   Place the broccoli, cauliflower, and onion on a second baking sheet and drizzle with olive oil. Sprinkle with 1/2 teaspoon salt and black pepper, toss to coat, then spread into an even layer. Place both baking sheets into your oven. Bake the tofu until dry and firm, about 20 minutes, and the vegetables until caramelized and tender, about 25 minutes. Flip the vegetables once halfway through, and rotate the top and bottom rack positions of the baking sheets. Set aside.

4   While the vegetables and tofu cook, prepare the dressing: In the bowl of a food processor or blender, place all of the dressing ingredients—tahini, lemon

juice, mint, parsley, salt, and pepper, and add 1/2 cup water. Blend until smooth.

5   a quick and easy tahini dressing being pulsed in a food processor for buddha bowls

6   Once the tofu is cooked, let cool slightly, and then place the tofu cubes in a bowl with 1/4 cup of the dressing and toss gently to coat. To assemble the bowls, scoop quinoa into a bowl, then top with the roasted vegetables, dressed tofu, and avocado, along with cucumber, almonds, and additional fresh mint and/or parsley as desired. Serve remaining dressing on the side and use as a dip or spoon over the top as desired.

7   tossing roasted crispy tofu with tahini dressing in a mixing bowl for buddha bowls

21. Red White and Blue Quinoa Fruit Salad

Prep Time: 20 Minutes

Cook Time: 0 Minutes

Servings: 4

Ingredients

For the Salad:

- 3/4 cup dry quinoa
- ounces fresh strawberries
- ounces fresh blueberries
- 1/2 cup toasted sliced almonds
- 1/4 cup fresh mint leaves julienned

For the Dressing:

- tablespoons honey use maple syrup or agave to make vegan
- 2 tablespoons lime juice
- 1/4 teaspoon salt

Instructions

1. Prepare quinoa according to package directions. Fluff and place in a large serving bowl, then let cool slightly. In a small bowl or measuring cup, stir together the dressing ingredients: honey, lime juice, and salt.

2. Trim and quarter the strawberries, then add them to the bowl along with the blueberries almonds and mint. Pour the dressing over the top, then toss gently to combine. Place in the refrigerator until ready to serve.

Prep Time: 20 Minutes

Cook Time: 40 Minutes

Servings: 4-6

Ingredients

- chicken drumsticks
- 4-5 bone-in, skin-on chicken thighs
- sea salt and ground pepper
- tablespoons olive oil
- 2 brown onions, peeled, cut into quarters through the root
- 2 tablespoons honey
- 2 tablespoons tomato paste
- zest and juice 1 lemon
- tablespoons purchased Moroccan spice mix
- cloves garlic, crushed
- 1½ cups pearl couscous (also called mograbieh)
- 3¾ cups chicken stock
- 3 bay leaves
- 1 cinnamon stick
- green or black olives

To serve

- tablespoons finely chopped pistachios
- 2 tablespoons finely chopped parsley
- Equipment: Large roasting dish or ovenproof baking dish big enough to take everything in a single layer (my tray is 42cm x 32cm x 3cm deep).

Instructions

1   Preheat the oven to 180°C fan bake.
2   Season the chicken with salt and pepper. Heat the oil in a large frying pan and cook the chicken skin side down until deeply golden brown. Transfer to the roasting dish. Don't wash the pan.
3   Add the onions to the pan and cook for 5 minutes, then add to the chicken. In a small bowl, stir the honey, tomato paste, lemon zest and juice, spice mix and garlic together, then tip into the pan and cook for 2 minutes. Stir in the couscous, stock, bay leaves and the cinnamon stick and bring to the boil.
4   Tip the mixture over the chicken and onions then distribute the couscous evenly so it's not all clumped together and flick off any that's on top of the chicken.

5   Cover tightly with foil and bake for 25 minutes. Uncover, scatter over the olives, then bake for a further 15 minutes, or until the chicken is fully cooked and the couscous is tender but still with a little bite. Scatter over the combined pistachios and parsley.

Prep Time: 15 Minutes

Cook Time: 25 Minutes

Servings: 2

Ingredients

Sauce:

- tablespoons gochujang (Korean red pepper paste)
- tablespoons honey
- 1 tablespoon soy sauce
- 1 tablespoon grated fresh ginger
- 2 cloves garlic, crushed
- 2 teaspoons sesame oil
- 2 teaspoons rice vinegar
- ½-1 teaspoon chilli flakes, to taste

To cook and serve

- 300 grams beef schnitzel, sliced into very thin strips
- sea salt and ground pepper
- vegetable oil
- 200 grams slim green beans, thinly sliced on the diagonal

- 1½ cups kimchi
- toasted sesame seeds and finely chopped coriander, to serve
- hot cooked noodles or rice, to serve

Instructions

1 Sauce: Mix all the ingredients together and set aside.

2 To cook and serve: Season the steak with salt and pepper. Heat a large frying pan with a little oil until searing hot. Add the steak in small batches and cook for 10-15 seconds. Transfer to a plate and cover to keep warm while you cook the remaining steak. Add a little more oil to the pan, add the beans and cook until lightly blistered. Add the kimchi and cook for 2 minutes, tossing together. Tip in the sauce and let it bubble up. Add the beef and resting juices and stir everything together.

3 Divide between bowls and top with the sesame seeds and coriander. Serve with noodles or rice.

Prep Time: 22 Minutes

Cook Time: 30 Minutes

Servings: 6

Ingredients

Meatballs:

- 1/3 cup panko breadcrumbs
- 150 grams ricotta or cottage cheese
- ½ cup freshly grated parmesan
- tablespoons milk or water
- 1 large egg
- 1 tablespoon dried oregano
- 2 cloves garlic, crushed
- 1 teaspoon sea salt
- finely grated zest 1 lemon
- 500 grams pork mince

To cook:

- 1 tablespoon each olive oil and butter
- 1 onion, thinly sliced
- 1 leek, thinly sliced

- cloves garlic, crushed
- teaspoons fennel seeds
- ¼-½ teaspoon chilli flakes
- sea salt and ground pepper
- 50 grams butter
- ¼ cup plain flour
- cups whole milk
- ½ cup cream
- 2 teaspoons Dijon mustard
- ½ teaspoon grated nutmeg
- 100 grams cheddar, grated, plus 30 grams extra for topping
- 60 grams gruyère, grated, plus 30 grams extra for topping
- ½ cup freshly grated parmesan, plus ½ cup extra for topping
- 500 grams macaroni or other small tube pasta
- Equipment: 6-cup capacity ovenproof baking dish.

Instructions

1. Preheat the oven to 180°C fan bake.
2. Meatballs: Combine all the ingredients except the pork in a large bowl and leave for 15 minutes. Add the

pork and mix until fully combined. Hands are good for this. Form into about 24 large walnut-sized meatballs. Heat a little oil in a large frying pan and, when hot, quickly brown the meatballs. They won't be fully cooked. Set aside. The meatballs can be browned several hours ahead of assembling.

3 To cook: Heat the oil and butter in a large frying pan and cook the onion, leek, garlic, fennel seeds and chilli with a good pinch of salt for 10 minutes or until very tender. Set aside.

4 Melt the 50 grams butter in a large saucepan and whisk in the flour until smooth. Cook over a low heat for 1 minute, then gradually whisk in the combined milk and cream, whisking continuously until smooth. Stir in the mustard and nutmeg and season well. Simmer for 5 minutes, stirring often. Remove from the heat and stir in the three cheeses until melted and smooth. Stir in three-quarters of the leek mixture and set the rest aside.

5 Cook the pasta in plenty of salted boiling water for 2 minutes less than the package instructions, then drain well. Combine the pasta with the sauce and tip into the baking dish. Nestle in the meatballs, then dot over the remaining leek mixture. Scatter over the

combined leftover three cheeses and bake for 25 minutes, until golden and bubbling around the edges.

Prep Time: 22 Minutes

Cook Time: 30 Minutes

Servings: 4

Ingredients

- 1½ teaspoons each ground cumin, coriander, turmeric, chilli powder, curry powder and sea salt
- skinless, boneless chicken thighs
- tablespoons olive oil
- 400ml tin coconut cream
- ½ cup each chicken stock and peanut butter
- 2 tablespoons kecap manis
- 1 tablespoon brown sugar
- 1 tablespoon rice wine vinegar
- finely grated zest and juice 1 large lime
- 1 teaspoon sesame oil
- cloves garlic, crushed
- 1 tablespoon grated fresh ginger
- small whole red chillies
- 1 stalk lemongrass, lightly bruised with a rolling pin
- ½ cup roasted peanuts, to garnish

Instructions

1 Preheat the oven to 180°C fan bake.

2 Combine all the spices and salt in a large bowl. Add the chicken and toss so each piece is well coated. Heat the oil in a large ovenproof frying pan over a medium heat and quickly brown the chicken on both sides. Transfer to a plate. Combine all the remaining ingredients except the chillies, lemongrass and peanuts in a large bowl. Tip into the frying pan and bring to the boil, crushing the peanut butter with a fork to amalgamate. Add the chicken and juices to the pan and turn to coat in the sauce. Nestle in the chillies and lemongrass. Bake for 35-40 minutes, or until the chicken is fully cooked. Top with the peanuts to serve.

Cook Time: 45 Minutes

Prep Time: 30 Minutes

Servings: 4

Ingredients

Paste:

- lemongrass stalks, tough outer skin removed, finely chopped
- 3cm piece ginger, chopped
- cloves garlic
- 2 red chillies

Curry

- tablespoons neutral oil
- lamb shanks, roughly 1.5 kilograms
- shallots, halved
- cardamom pods, toasted
- 1 teaspoon each ground cumin and coriander
- ½ teaspoon ground turmeric
- 2 cups chicken stock
- 400ml tin coconut cream

- 1 makrut lime leaf

- 2 cinnamon sticks

- 2 star anise

- 1 tablespoon each tamarind paste and brown sugar

- 1 teaspoon sea salt

- 2 dried red chillies

- 80 grams desiccated coconut

- 1 tablespoon each lime juice and brown sugar

Instructions

1. Preheat the oven to 160°C regular bake.
2. PASTE: Blitz all the ingredients in a food processor.
3. CURRY: In a large ovenproof casserole dish, heat the oil over a medium heat. Brown the shanks on all sides, then set aside. Reduce the heat to low, add the paste the pan and fry for 3 minutes, stirring regularly. Add the shallots, cardamom pods and ground spices and fry for a further 2 minutes. Add the lamb, stock, coconut cream, lime leaf, cinnamon, star anise, tamarind, brown sugar, sea salt and chillies and bring to a simmer. Cover and cook in the oven for 3 hours, or until the meat is tender. Toast the coconut in a frying pan over a medium heat until golden, then set

aside. Remove the lamb from the curry, set aside and cover with foil. Increase the oven to 180°C regular bake. Add the coconut, lime juice and sugar to the curry and season with salt. Return to the oven for 15 minutes, uncovered. Once thickened, return the shanks to the curry and return to the oven briefly to warm through.

Cook Time: 45 Minutes

Prep Time: 30 Minutes

Servings: 4

Ingredients

- ½ cup plain flour
- sea salt and ground pepper
- 600 grams skinless, boneless Rangitikei chicken breasts, cut thinly on an angle into ½ cm-thick slices
- tablespoons each olive oil and butter
- 340-gram jar artichoke quarters, drained
- 1 cup white wine
- tablespoons capers, well drained
- 2 cloves garlic, crushed
- finely grated zest 1 lemon
- pinch chilli flakes
- 2 packed cups baby spinach leaves
- 200 grams crème fraîche
- 250 grams pappardelle, cooked and hot

- 2 tablespoons parsley, finely chopped

Instructions

1   Season the flour and coat the chicken, shaking off the excess flour.

2   Heat half the oil and butter in a large frying pan and fry the chicken in batches until cooked through, adding the remaining oil and butter between batches. Transfer to a plate and cover to keep warm.

3   Add the artichokes, wine, capers, garlic, zest and chilli flakes to the pan and let it bubble up and reduce a little. Add the spinach, turning to wilt. Season, then stir in the crème fraîche until melted and bubbling. Add the chicken with the resting juices, then stir in the pasta, turning to combine. Add the parsley and serve in warm shallow bowls.

Cook Time: 15 Minutes

Prep Time: 45 Minutes

Servings: 6

Ingredients

Marinade:

- cloves garlic, crushed
- finely grated zest
- 1 large lemon
- tablespoons lemon juice
- 1 tablespoon each cumin seeds, ground coriander, dried oregano and dried mint
- 2 teaspoons smoked paprika
- 1 teaspoon each ground cinnamon and chilli flakes
- 2 teaspoons sea salt
- ground pepper, to taste
- 1/3 cup olive oil
- skinless, boneless chicken thighs (about 1.2 kilograms)

To cook

- red capsicums, quartered, then each piece cut in half
- red onions, cut into quarters and pieces separated
- large fresh bay leaves
- Equipment: 4 x 35cm metal skewers, wire rack and large roasting dish or lipped baking tray.

Instructions

1 MARINADE: Combine all the ingredients except the chicken in a large bowl. Add the chicken and turn to coat well. Cover and chill for 1-8 hours.

2 TO COOK: Fold the short sides of the thighs together. Thread the thighs, alternating with pieces of capsicum and onion and the bay leaves, onto two skewers, packing them tightly and ensuring both skewers go through each piece of chicken and veg.

3 Preheat the oven to 200°C fan bake.

4 Place the wire rack over the roasting dish and add enough water to cover the base of the dish. Place the skewers on top of the rack and roast for 20 minutes. Flip them over, drizzle with a little oil and cook for a further 20 minutes, or until fully cooked. Cooking time will depend on the size of the thighs. Transfer to a serving board and spoon over any juices in the dish.

Cook Time: 30 Minutes

Prep Time: 60 Minutes

Servings: 4

Ingredients

- 1 kilogram Agria potatoes, peeled and sliced 1cm thick
- 1 large brown onion, thinly sliced
- 400-gram tin crushed Italian tomatoes
- ½ cup white wine
- cloves garlic, crushed
- sea salt and ground pepper
- 1 Rangitikei Free Range whole chicken
- 1 large lemon, halved
- bunch woody herbs, use any combination of rosemary, thyme and bay leaves
- 1 tablespoon olive oil

Olive and Pistachio Dressing

- ½ cup roughly chopped green olives
- ¼ cup pistachios, chopped

- ¼ cup each mint and parsley leaves, finely chopped
- cloves garlic, crushed
- 2 teaspoons finely grated lemon zest
- 1 tablespoon lemon juice
- 1/3 cup olive oil
- ½-1 teaspoon honey, to taste

Instructions

1. Preheat the oven to 170°C fan bake. Toss the potatoes, onion, tomatoes, wine and garlic in a large bowl and season. Spread evenly in a roasting dish and bake for 30 minutes.

2. Season the chicken cavity and squeeze in the lemon, then add the squeezed halves and herbs. Tie the legs with kitchen string and tuck the wings under. Place on top of the potatoes. Brush with oil and season well. Roast for 1½ hours, or until fully cooked.

3. Dressing: Combine all the ingredients and season well.

4. To serve: Spoon over some dressing, serving the rest separately.

Cook Time: 10 Minutes

Prep Time: 4hrs,20 Minutes

Servings: 6

Ingredients

- black pepper
- 1 1/2 cups shredded part-skim shredded mozzarella cheese divided
- 1/2 cup freshly grated Parmesan cheese about 1 1/4 ounces
- jars good-quality red pasta sauce (24-ounce jars) divided
- ounces 2 teaspoons extra-virgin olive oil
- ounces sliced cremini baby bella mushrooms
- 1 small red onion or yellow onion, diced
- 1 red bell pepper cored and diced
- cups lightly packed fresh baby spinach about 4 ounces
- 2 cloves garlic minced
- ounces part-skim ricotta cheese (1 container)
- 1 large egg
- 1/2 teaspoon kosher salt

- 1/2 teaspoon uncooked whole wheat ziti or penne noodles, or swap a similar short, hollow noodle Chopped fresh basil or parsley, optional for serving

Instructions

1 Heat the olive oil in large nonstick skillet over medium-high heat. Once hot, add the mushrooms and onions, and sauté until they're beginning to brown and soften, about 6 minutes. Add the bell pepper and cook for 3 minutes, then add the garlic. Add the spinach a few handfuls at a time, stirring and cooking until spinach wilts and the garlic smells fragrant, 1 to 2 additional minutes. Remove from the heat and set aside.

2 In a medium bowl, combine the ricotta, egg, salt, and pepper, until combined. Stir in 1/2 cup mozzarella and Parmesan.

3 Generously coat the inside of a 4-quart or larger slow cooker with cooking spray. Spread a thin layer of sauce on the bottom, then top with half of the pasta noodles. Pour 2 cups sauce over the top and spread it into an even layer with the back of a spoon or spatula.

Dollop half of the ricotta mixture on top, then sprinkle with half of the sautéed vegetables.

4   Repeat the layers: remaining noodles, 2 cups of sauce, remaining ricotta, and remaining vegetables. Pour the remaining sauce on top and spread evenly. Cover and cook on low for 3 to 4 hours or on high for 1 to 2 hours. Check at the 3 (on low) or 1 (on high) hour mark to ensure the pasta does not over cook. To check for doneness, use a fork to pull a "test" noodle from the center of the slow cooker. Once it is tender, the pasta is done.

5   Sprinkle the top with the remaining 1 cup mozzarella cheese. Cover, turn the heat to high, and cook until the cheese is melted, 5 to 10 minutes. Serve warm, topped with chopped fresh basil or parsley.